LUKE LEARNS ABOUT "INSIDE THE BODY"

Copyright: Kerrice Accarias
First Published: 06-01-2018
Published in: Australia
ISBN: 978-0-9954456-8-0

Dedicated to my husband
and
All the Children of the World.

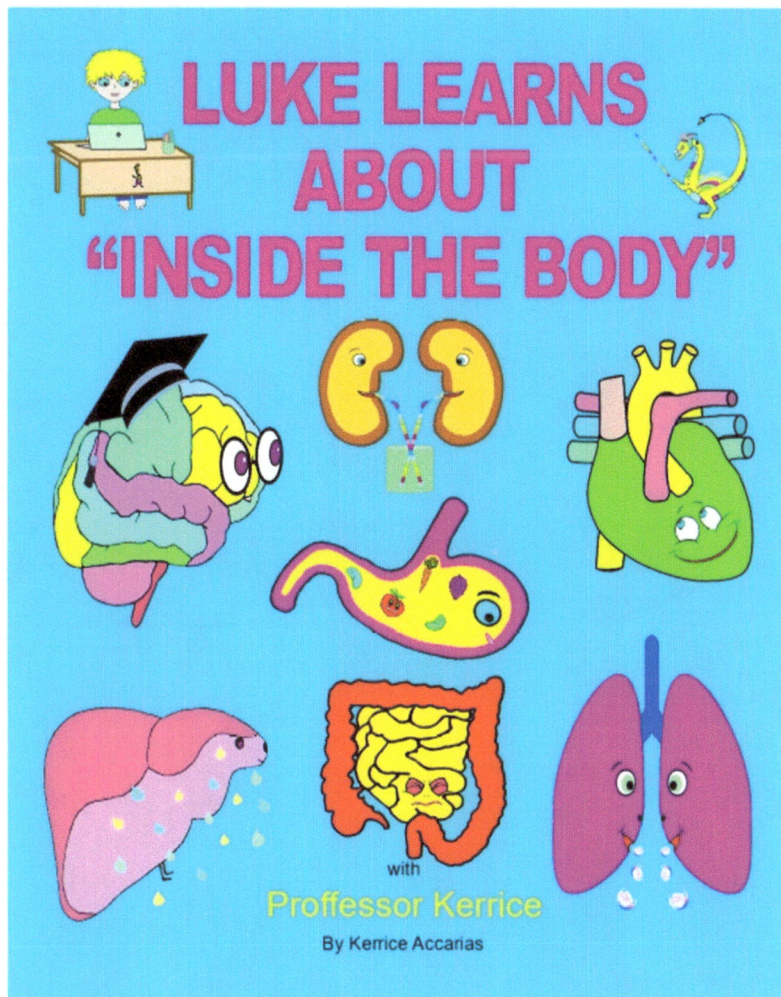

Written
&
Illustrations
by
Kerrice Accarias

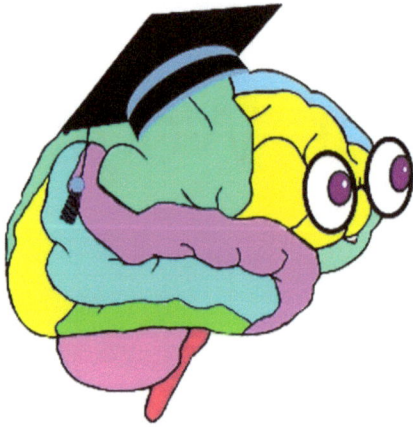

BRAIN

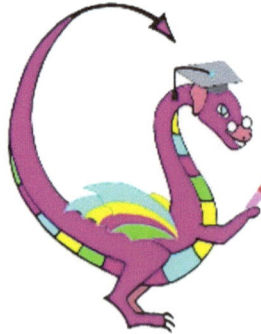

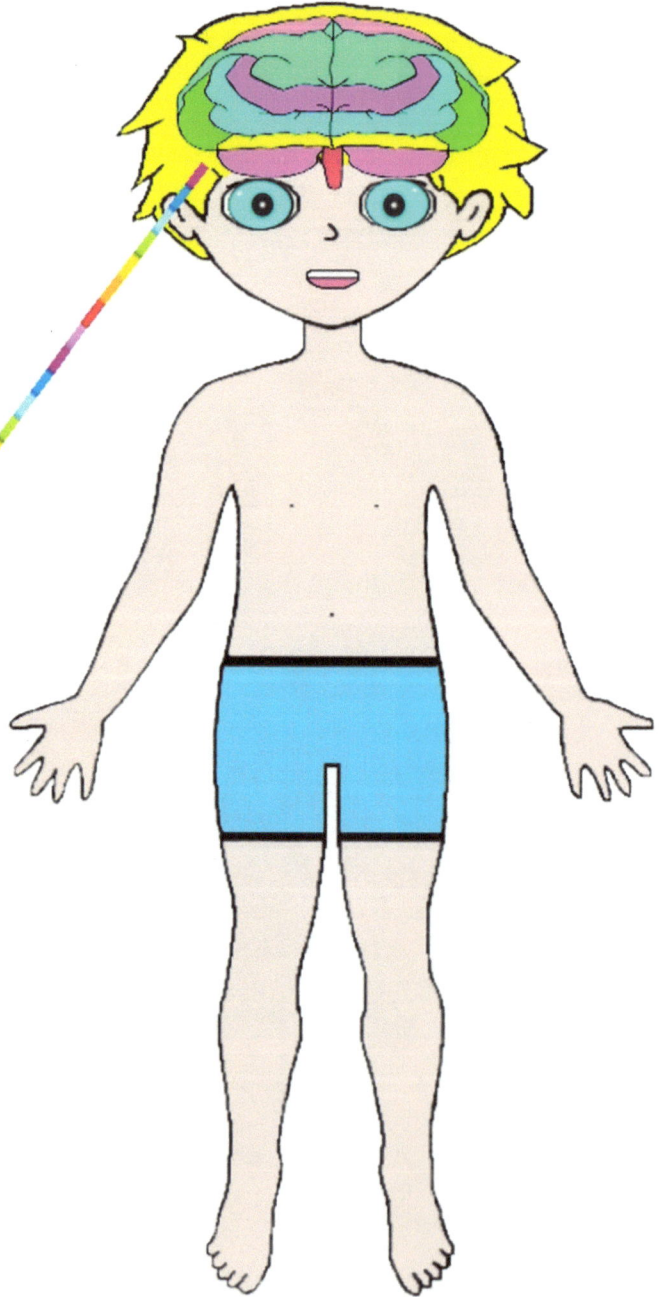

BRAIN

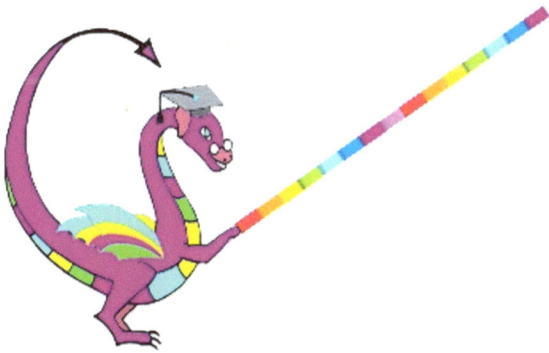

Luke has a **BRAIN**
It's a thinking machine.
Knowing 1 apple is red
And another is green.
Like a computer
It knows many things.
A dog has 4 legs
And a bird has wings.

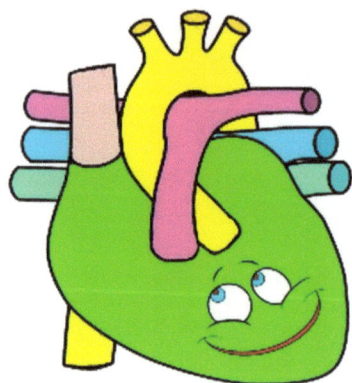

HEART

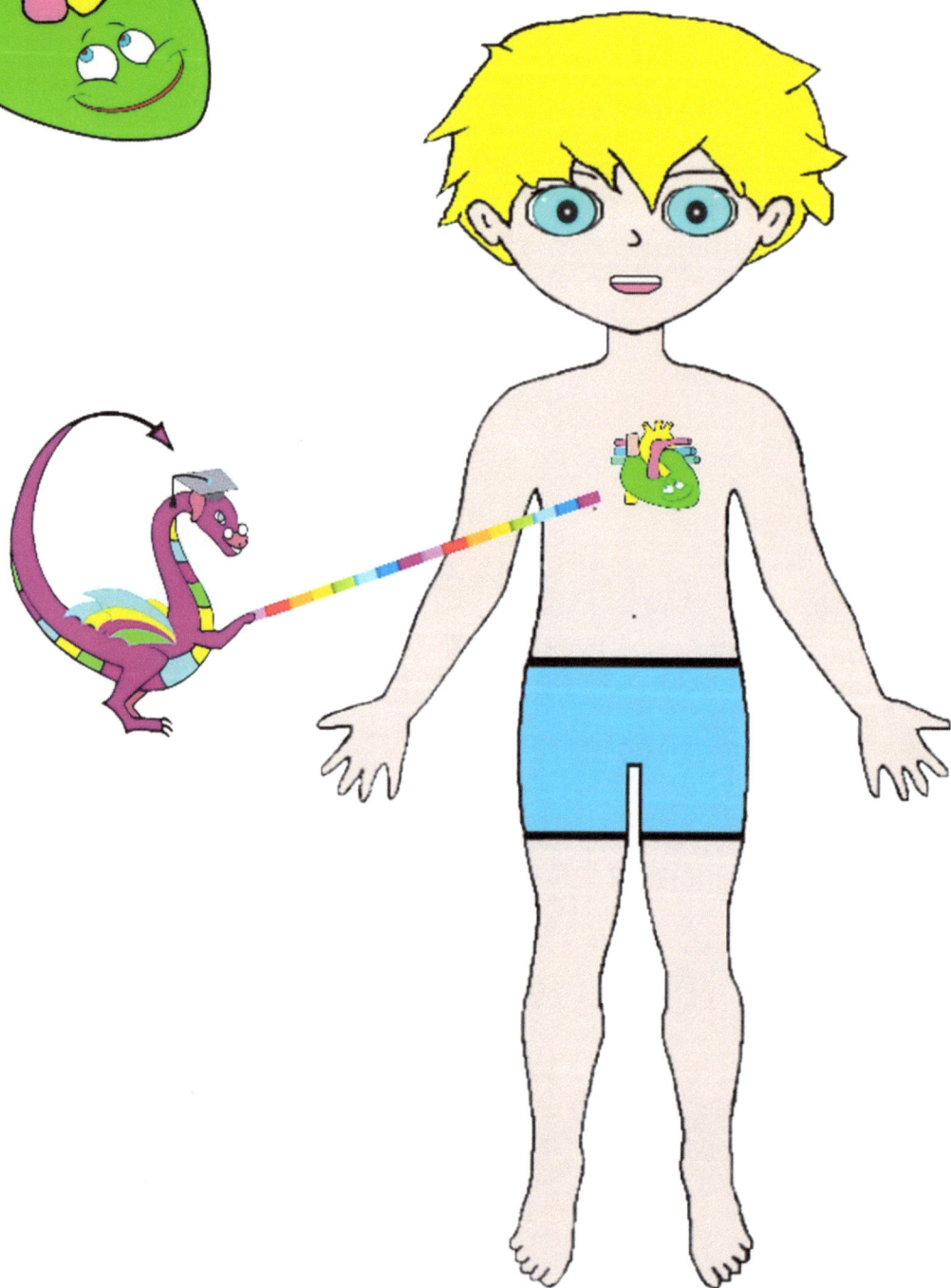

HEART

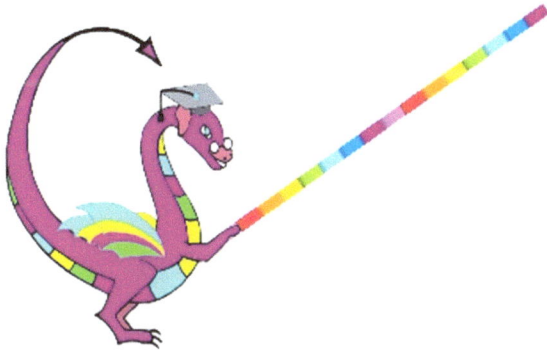

Luke has a **HEART**
It's tough and strong.
He keeps it pumping
Through movement and song.
Luke's heart is happy
When the blood flows through.
His heart needs exercise
and love helps too.

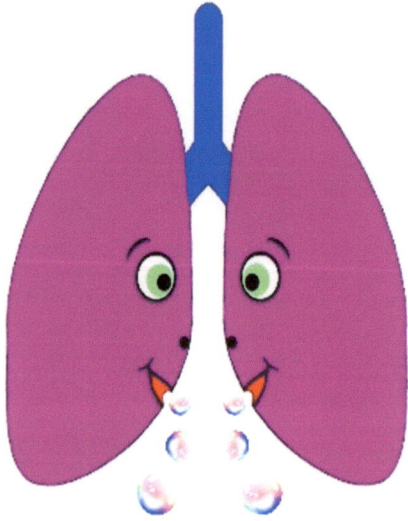

LUNGS

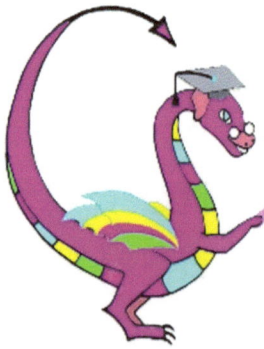

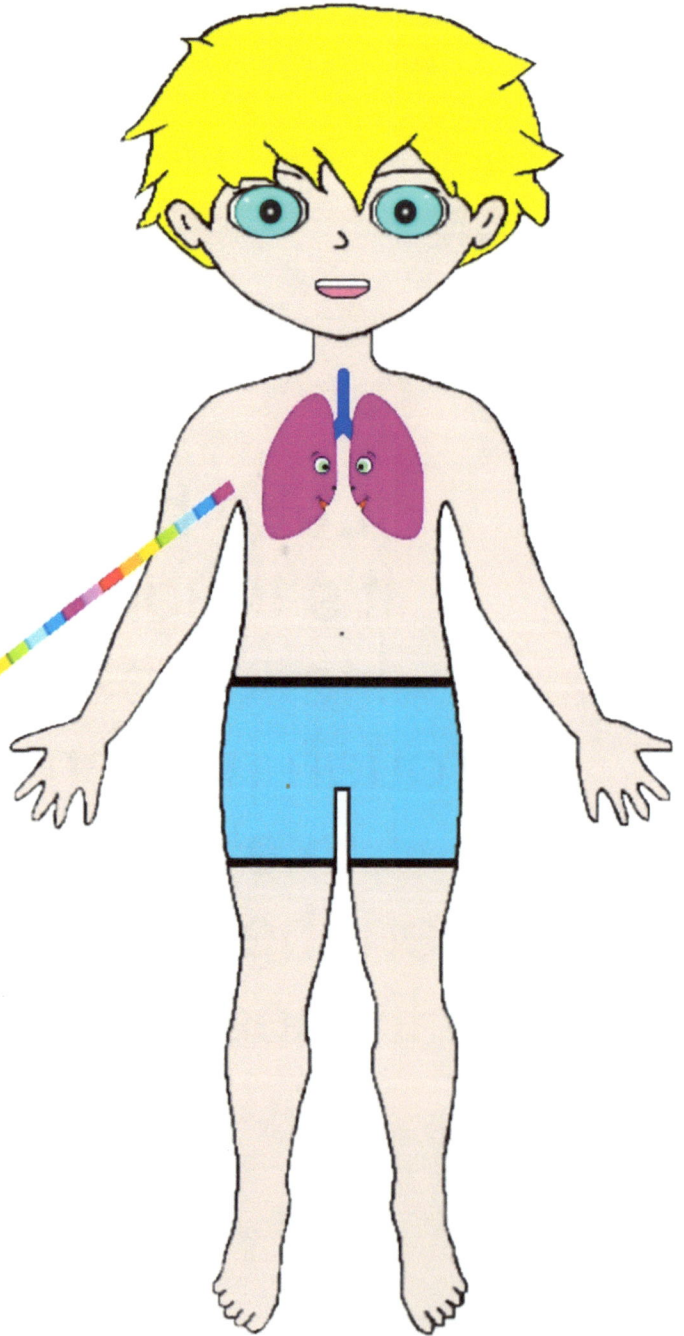

LUNGS

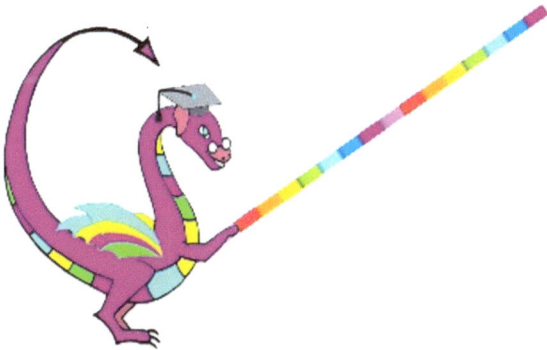

Luke has **Lungs**
They are filled with air.
He blows bubbles
From the air in there.
Running and jumping
And singing a song.
Luke needs fresh air
To keep them strong.

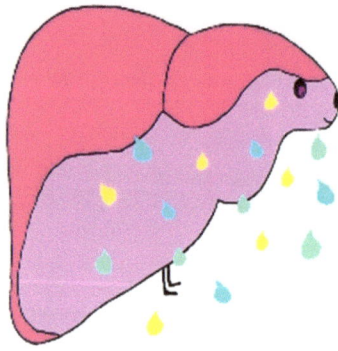 # LIVER

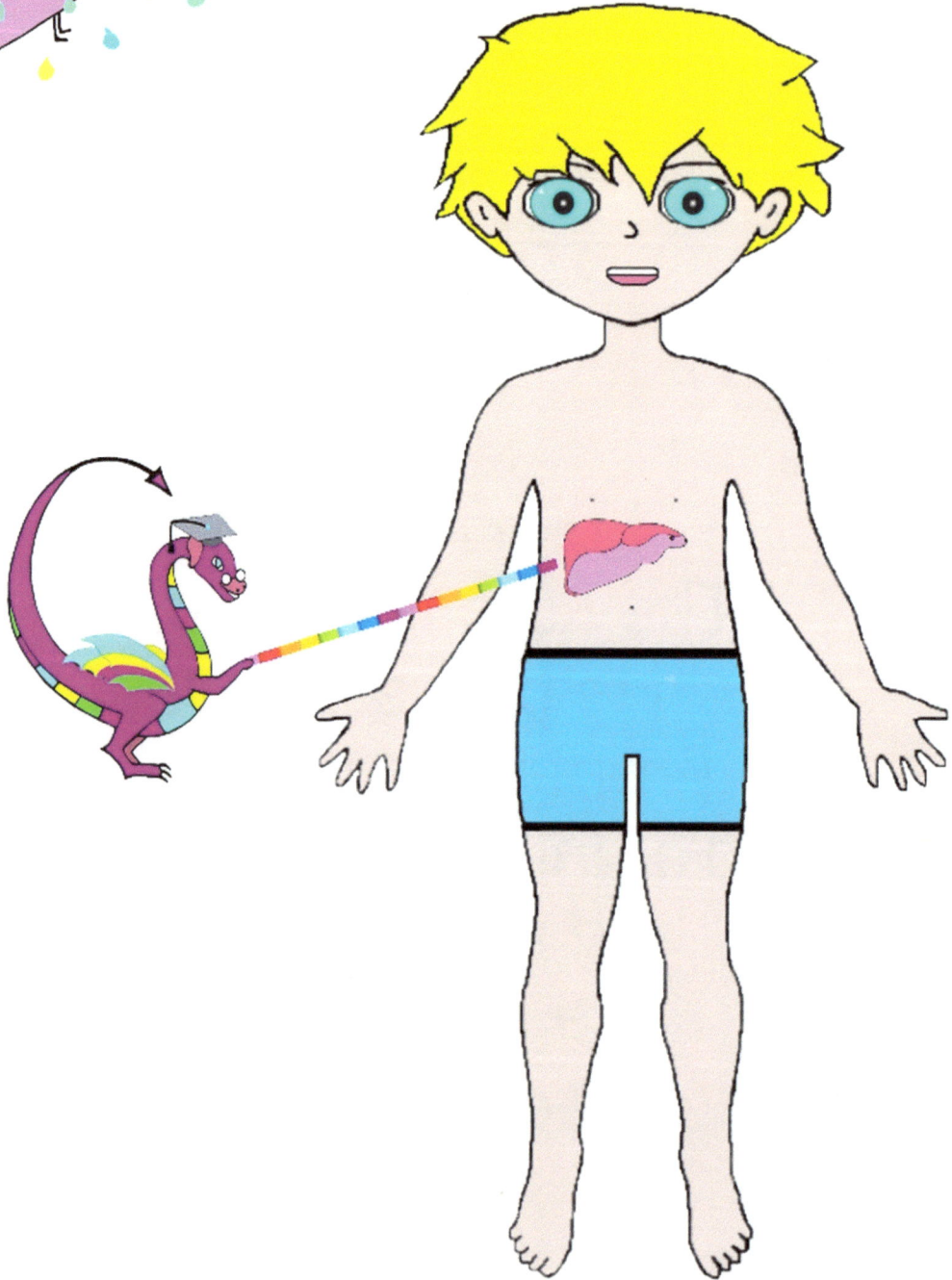

LIVER

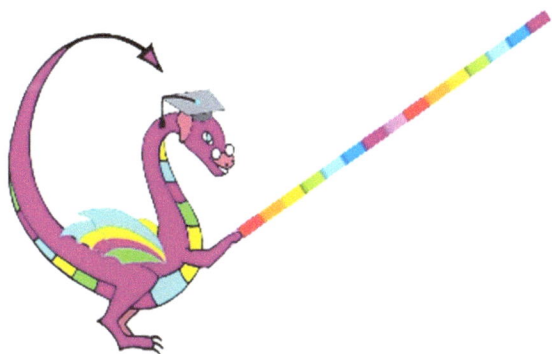

Luke has a **LIVER**
It cleans his blood.
Bad food and drink
Makes it flow like mud.
So being active
And eating right.
Helps his Liver
Feel healthy and light.

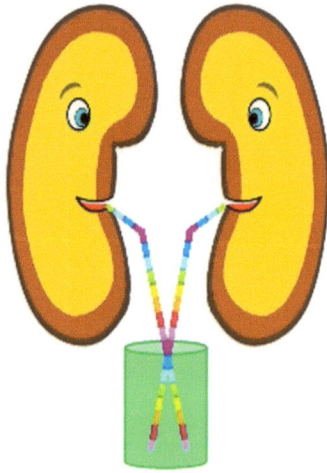

KIDNEYS

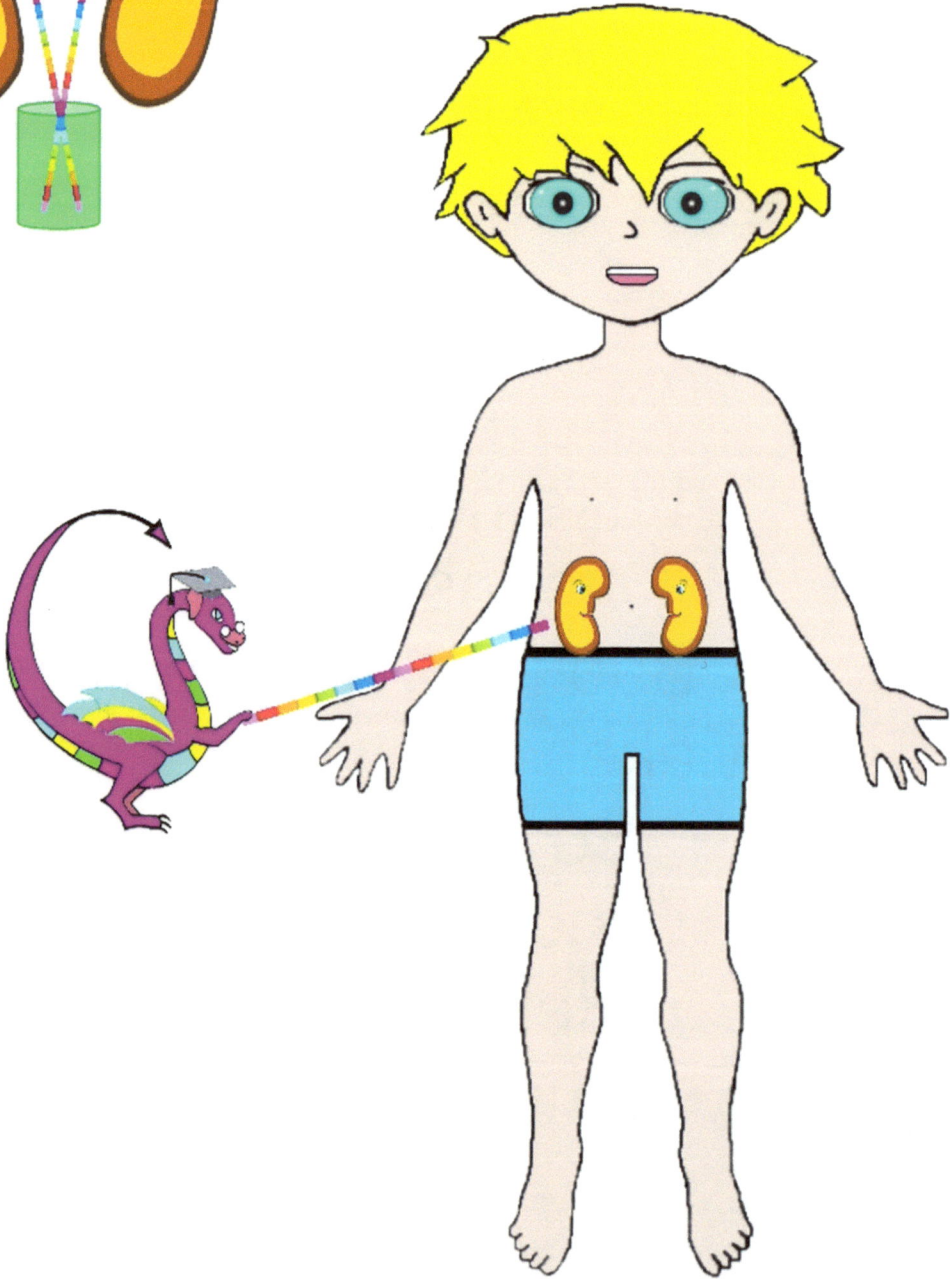

KIDNEYS

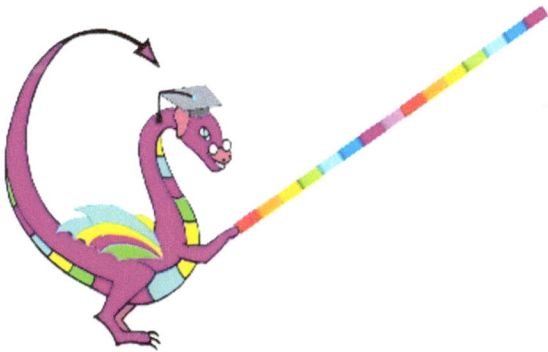

Luke has **KIDNEYS**
Shaped like beans.
Working together
As cleaning machines.
Luke drinks water
Each night and day.
Keeping them healthy
Washing baddies away.

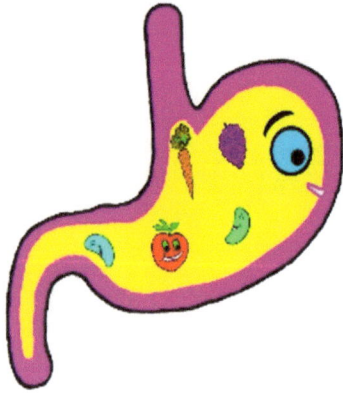

STOMACH

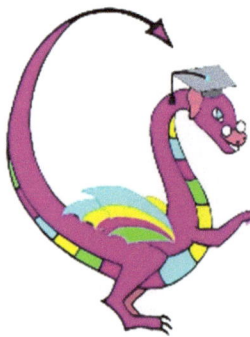

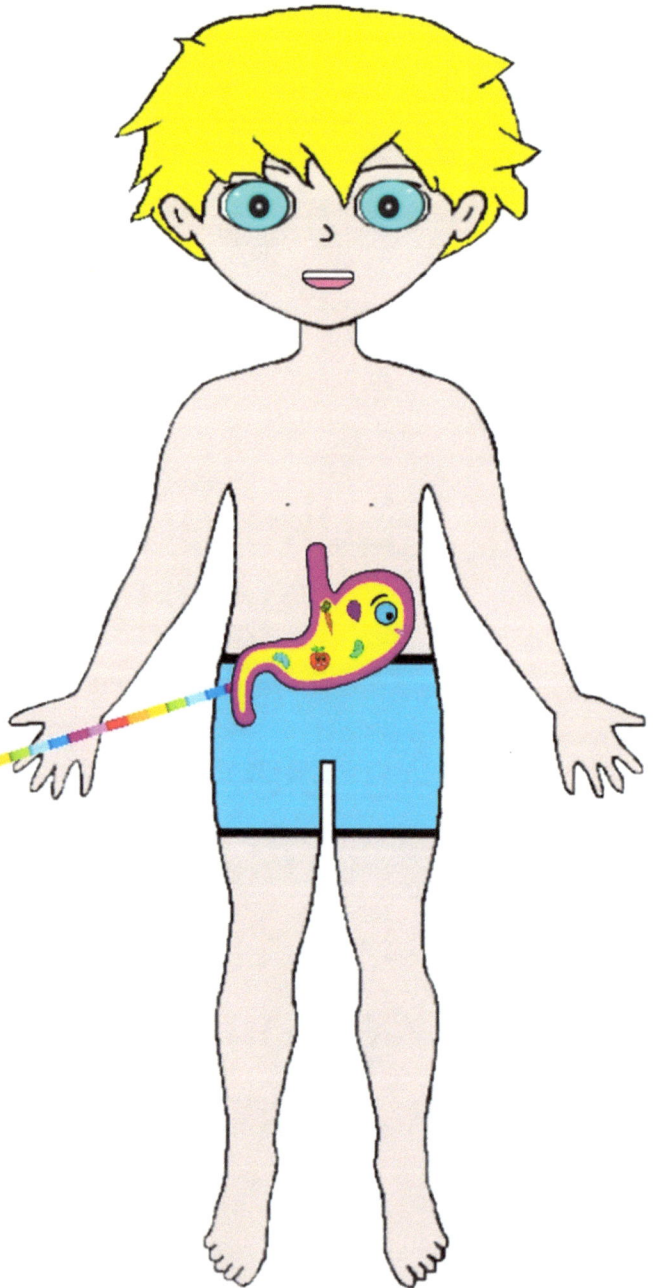

STOMACH

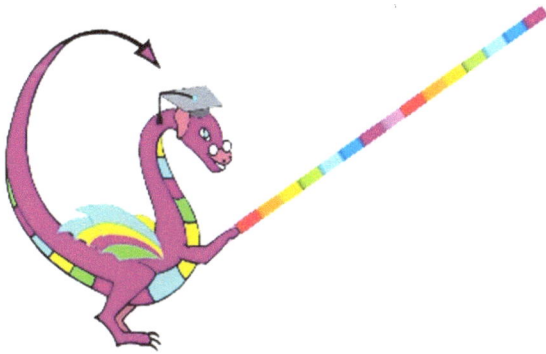

Luke has a STOMACH
Needing good food.
When Luke eats well
He's in a good mood.
Lots of fruit and veggies
A little fish and meat.
And only sometimes
A small healthy treat.

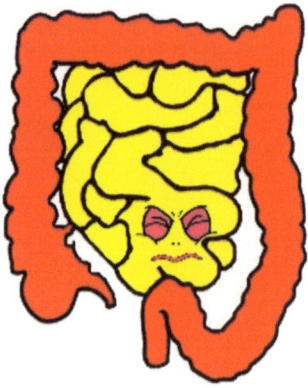 # INTESTINES

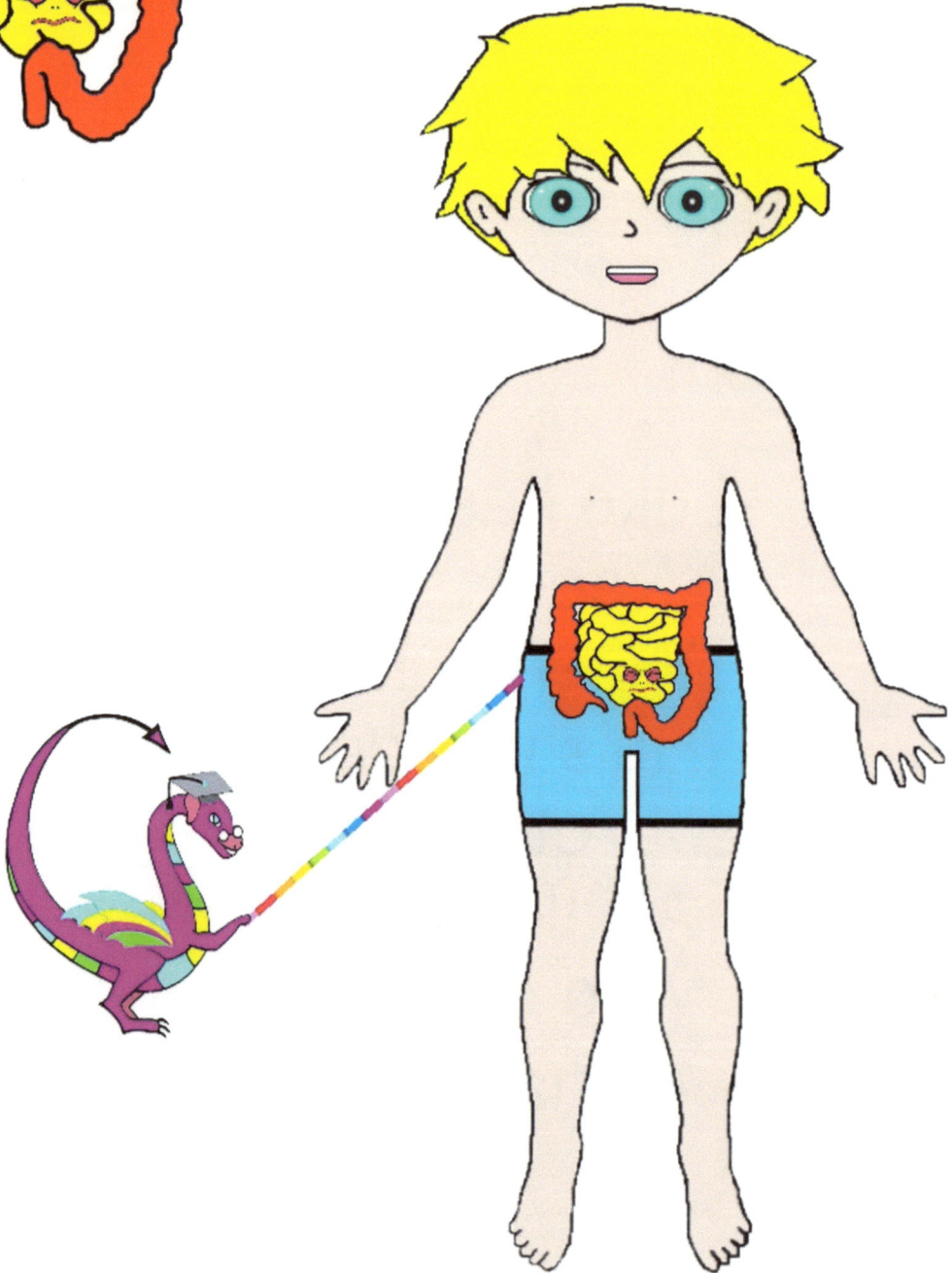

INTESTINES

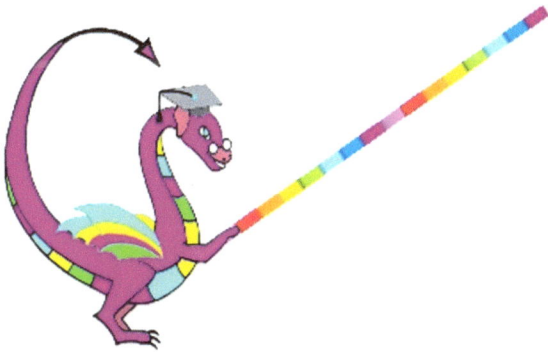

Luke has **INTESTINES**
They're long and lumpy.
When the food is eaten
It gets big and bumpy.
Good oils and fiber
Helps food slide through.
His Tract is now happy
And Luke is too.

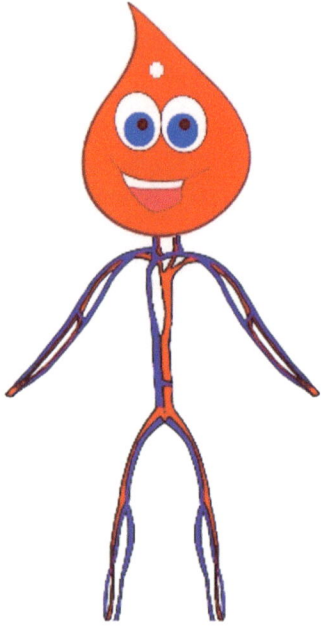

VEINS

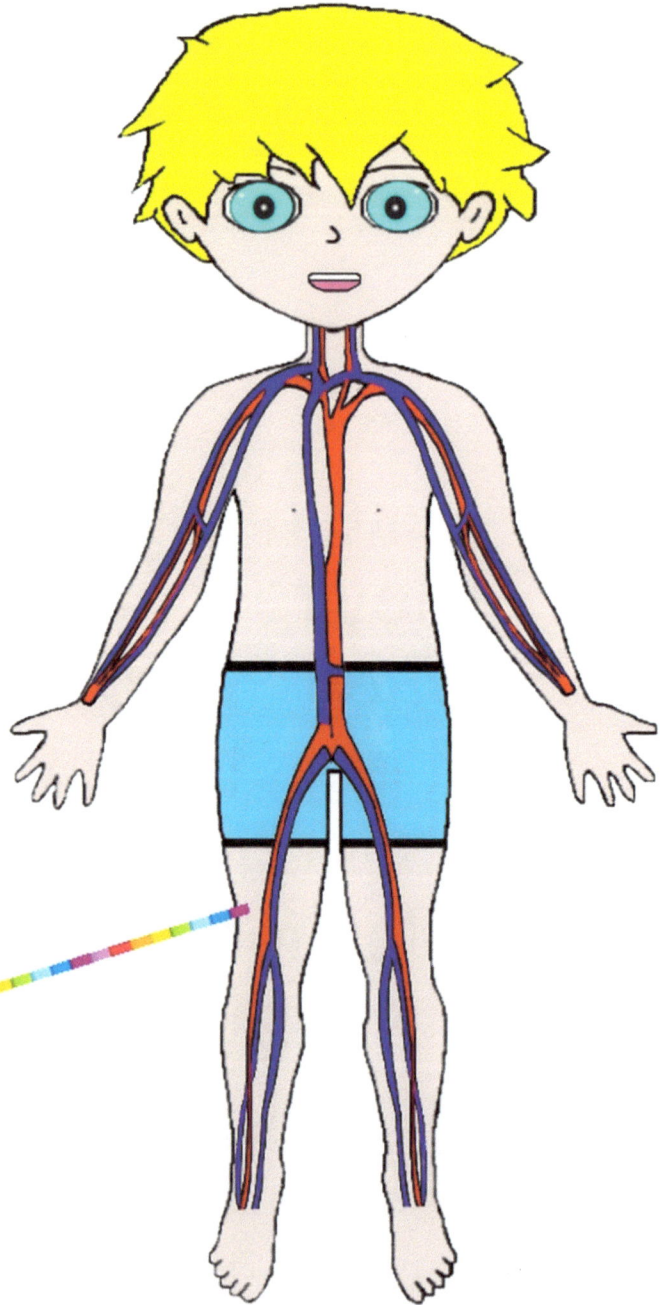

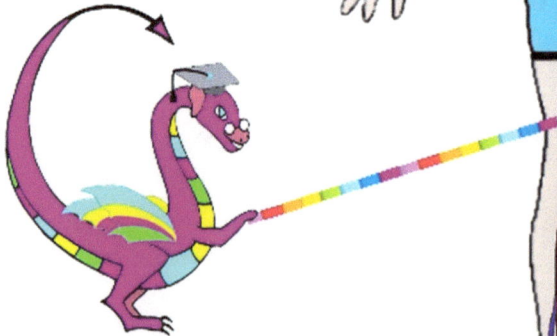

VEINS

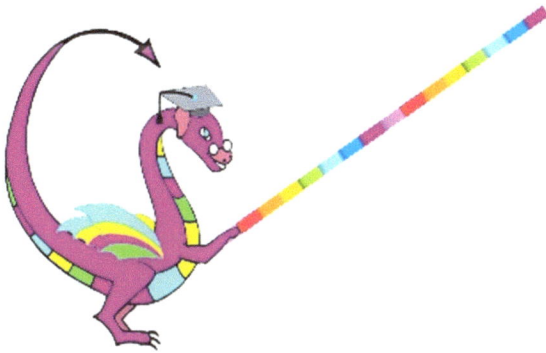

Luke has **VEINS**
Where blood flows through.
They're thin and long
Kate has them too.
With exercise and play
It flows like a stream.
All through the body
Veins work as a team.

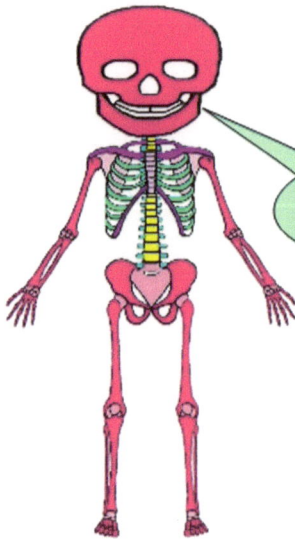

BONES

206 BONES

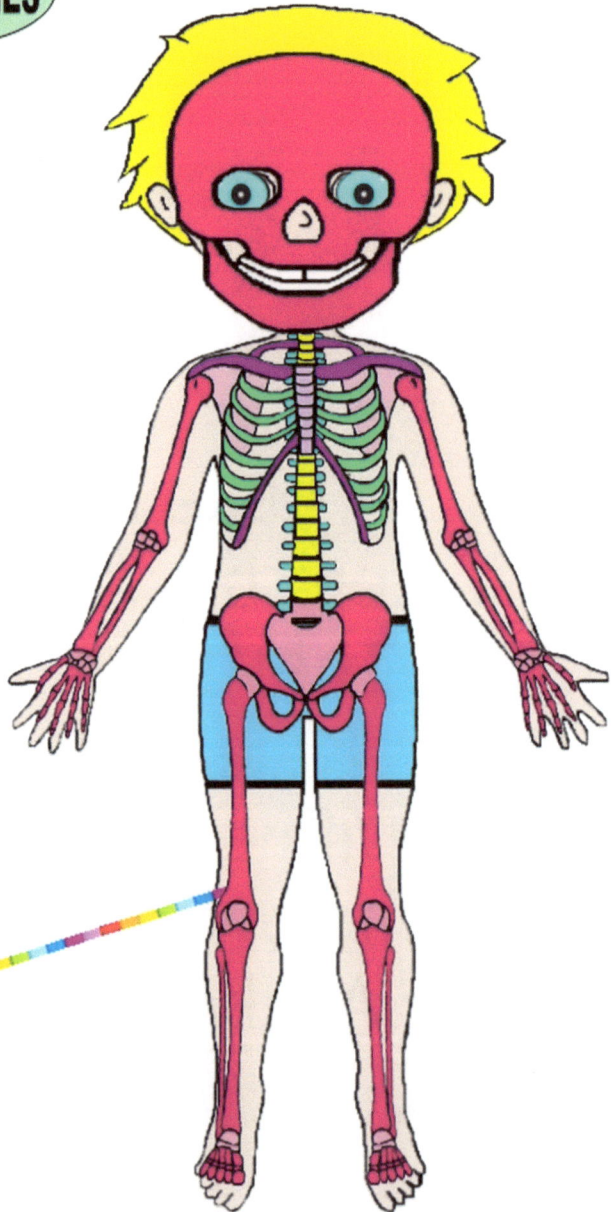

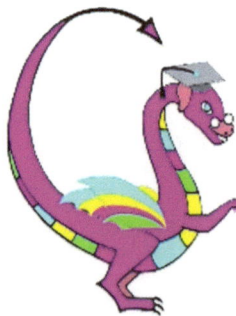

BONES

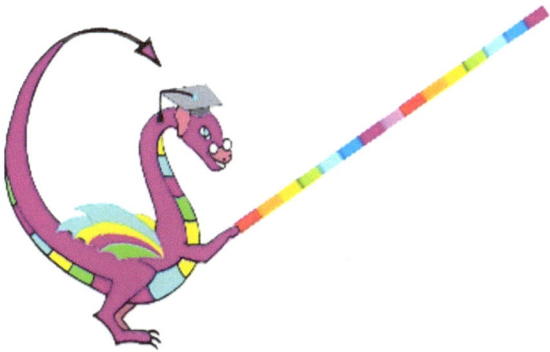

Luke has **BONES**
They are hard to break.
He keeps them strong
Not soft like a snake.
Lifting and moving
Eating yogurt and cheese.
Getting some sun
Keeps them healthy with ease.

INSIDE THE BODY

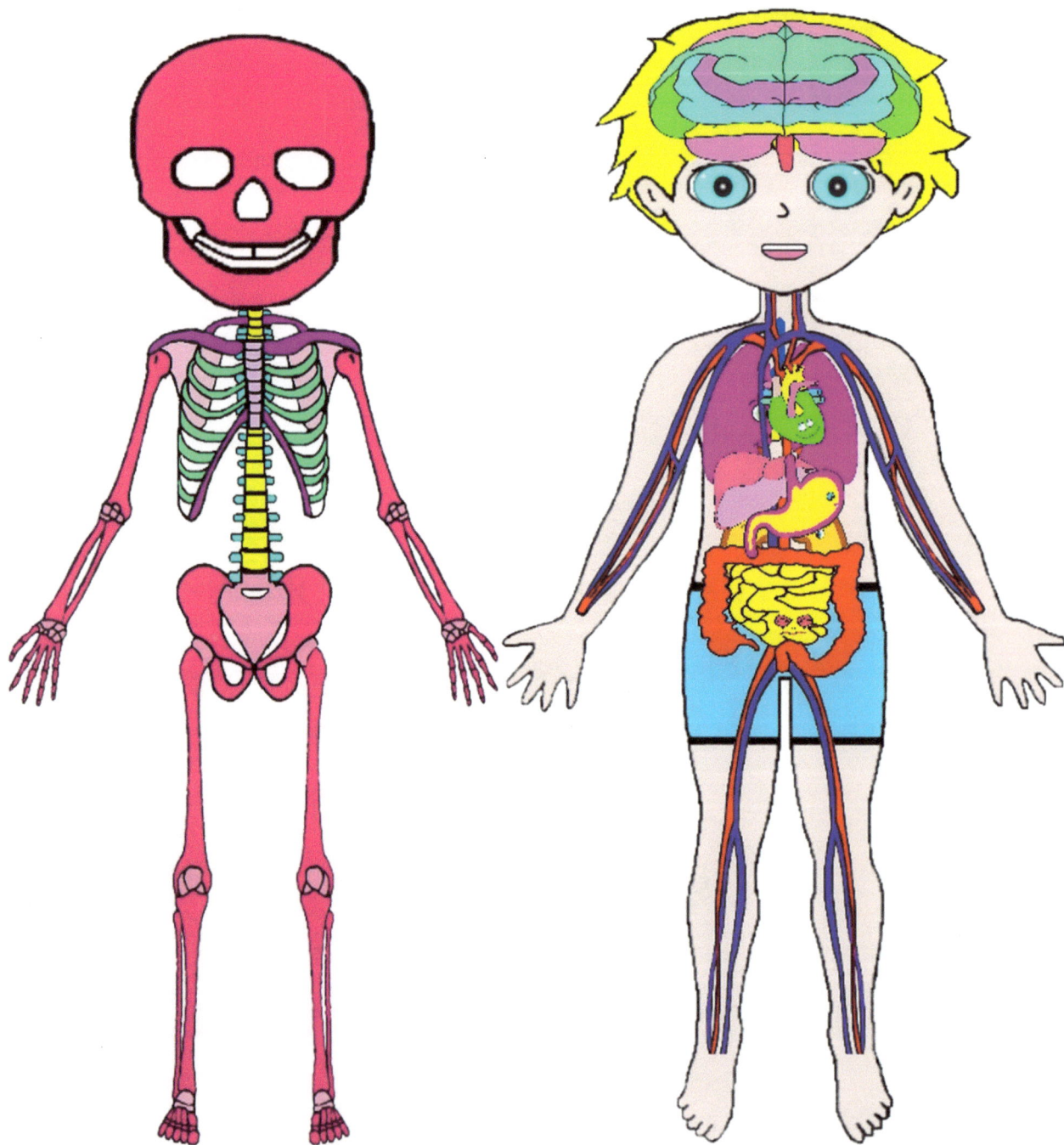

INSIDE THE BODY

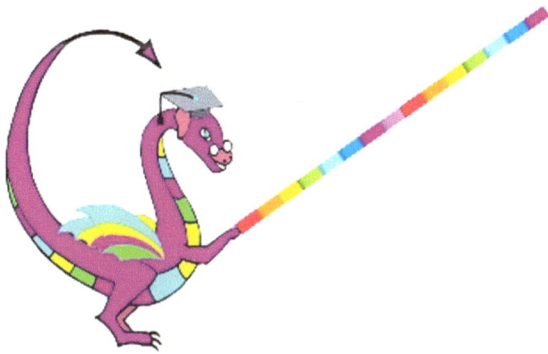

INSIDE THE BODY
Is a working machine.
All working together
To keep healthy and clean.
You must eat well
Exercise and be kind.
So you'll be happy
In Body and Mind.

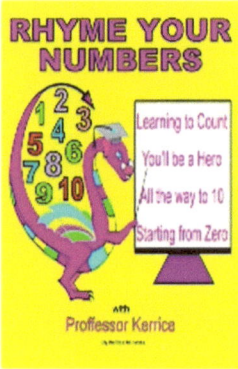

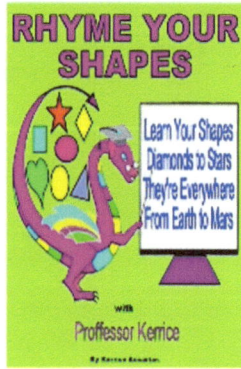

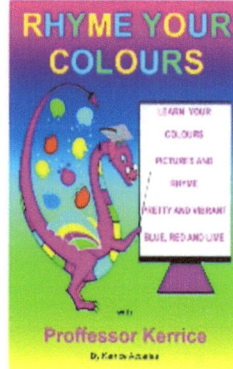

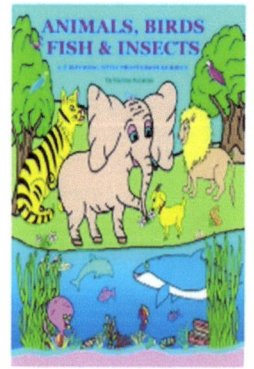

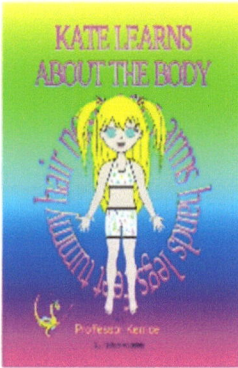

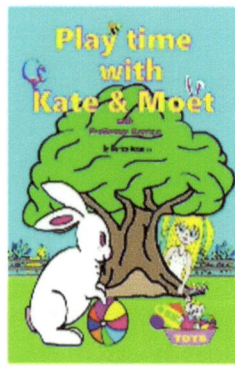

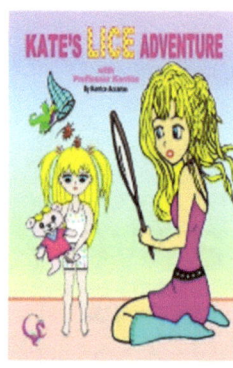

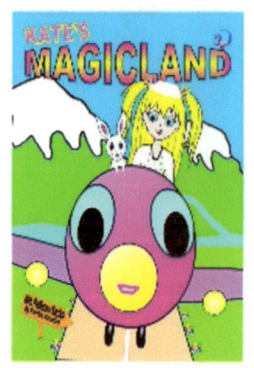

NEXT BOOK

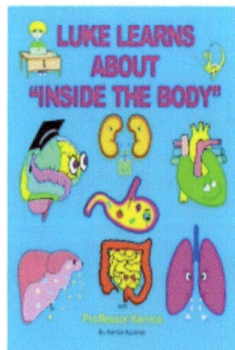

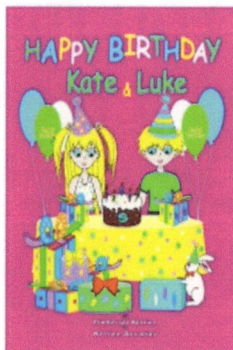